Your In
Vegeta

Discover Healthy and _____ ____pes and
Change ____ Lifestyle

America Best Recipes

Table of Contents

Breakfast
Roasted Baby Eggplant
Servings: 16 halves

Ingredients

8 baby eggplant 2 Tbsp olive oil

1 tsp Wild Fennel Pollen (optional) 1 tsp kosher or sea salt

1 tsp freshly ground pepper to serve:

1/3 cup ricotta cheese

2 Tbsp extra virgin olive oil Freshly ground pepper Kosher or sea salt to taste

Instructions

Wash the eggplant and cut them into halves. Place on a cookie sheet cut side up. Drizzle with the olive oil and then sprinkle with the fennel pollen (if using), salt and pepper.

Bake in a 350 degree (F) oven for about 45 minutes, or until softened and lightly browned. Remove from the oven and let cool slightly. Serve warm or at room temperature.

Right before serving top with about a teaspoon of ricotta cheese per half. Sprinkle with freshly cracked peppercorns (pink or mixed if you have them) and just a few grains of salt. Drizzle with a good quality extra virgin olive oil.

Based on my experiments, the best way to eat them is similar to an artichoke leaf. Just sink your teeth in and pull, scraping off all of the delicious filling, and leaving the tough skin behind.

Nutrition Info

Serving Size: half an eggplant Calories: 44 Fat: 4g Carbohydrates: 1g Fiber: 1g Protein: 1g

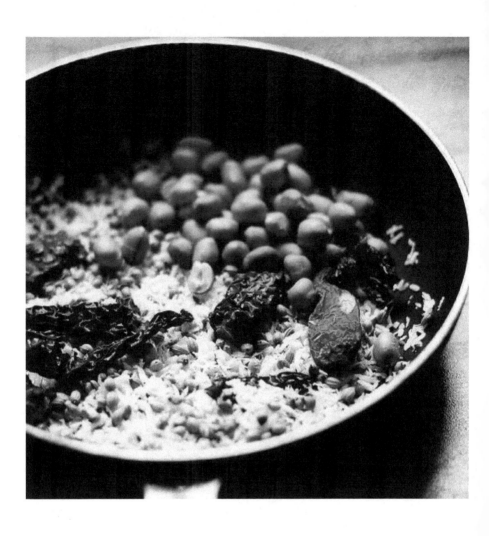

Moroccan Roasted Green Beans

Give boring green beans another chance with these delicious Moroccan Spiced Roasted Green Beans! Keto, Atkins, Paleo and Whole 30 approved!

Servings: 6 servings

Ingredients

6 cups raw green beans, trimmed 1 tsp kosher salt

1/2 tsp ground black pepper

1 Tbsp Ras el Hanout seasoning 2 Tbsp olive oil

Instructions

Toss the green beans, olive oil and seasonings together and spread out on a large cookie sheet or roasting pan.

Roast at 400 degrees (F) for 20 minutes. Remove from the oven and stir.

Return to the oven and roast an additional 10 minutes. Remove and serve warm or chilled.

Nutrition Info

73 calories 5g fat 4g net carbs 2g protein

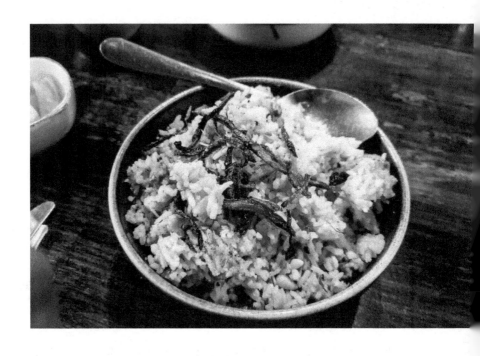

Scrambled Eggs with Cheese

Prep time: 10 min Cooking Time: 10 min Serve: 2

Ingredients

4 eggs

1 cup goat cheese, grated

2 tablespoons coconut oil

Salt and pepper to taste

2 tablespoons coconut milk

½ tablespoon butter

1 cup of water

Instructions

Spray a small, heat-proof bowl with coconut oil.

Break the 4 eggs into the bowl.

Add the milk, salt and pepper, and beat with a fork until more or less uniform.

Add the butter.

Put 1 cup of water in the Instant Pot and add the trivet.

Set the bowl on the trivet, and close the Instant Pot and its steam vent.

Set the Instant Pot to Steam at Low Pressure for 7 minutes. The Instant Pot will start chugging away, heating the water, and then counting down from 7 minutes.

Release the pressure immediately after the timer is down and open the Instant Pot. The eggs should look mostly cooked.

Serve and enjoy.

Nutrition Facts

Calories 342, Total Fat 31g, Saturated Fat 21.1g, Cholesterol 342mg , Sodium 174mg, Total Carbohydrate 1.9g, Dietary Fiber 0.3g , Total Sugars 1.5g, Protein 15.7g

Caramelized Banana Dark Chocolate Oatmeal

Prep time: 10 min Cooking Time: 10 min Serve: 2

Ingredients

2 cups water

1 cup rolled oats

Olive oil

Salt

½ tablespoon butter

1 medium banana, sliced

2 tablespoons dark chocolate chips

Instructions

Prepare the Instant Pot with 2 cups of water and the steamer basket.

In a small heat-proof bowl or mug, add the oats, water, salt and butter.

Close and lock lid and set the valve to "Sealing".

Pressure Cook for 3 minutes at High Pressure.

While oats are cooking, spray a small non-stick skillet with olive oil. Add sliced bananas in a single layer and cook over medium heat until caramelized, about 3 minutes per side.

Disengage the ─Keep Warm‖ mode or unplug the cooker and open when the pressure indicator has gone down for 7 to 15 minutes.

Spoon oatmeal into a bowl and top with caramelized bananas and chocolate chips.

Nutrition Facts

Calories 245, Total Fat 5.2g, Saturated Fat 1.8g,Cholesterol 0mg, Sodium 10mg, Total Carbohydrate

46.2g, Dietary Fiber 5.7g ,Total Sugars 11.6g, Protein 6.5g

Vegetable Muffins

Prep time: 10 min Cooking Time: 10 min Serve: 2

Ingredients

1/2 bell pepper, red

1 spring onion

4 eggs

1/2 handful kale

1/4 cup goat cheese

¼ teaspoon salt and pepper

1 teaspoon hot sauce

Cooking spray

1 cup of water

1 teaspoon scallions

Instructions

Spray 6 ovenproof custard cups with non-stick cooking spray.

In a large bowl, whisk the eggs, salt and pepper, cheese until just blended. Evenly divide the kale, bell pepper, spring onion, sauce and scallions among the custard cups. Pour the egg mixture over the veggies.

Pour 1 cup of water into the Instant Pot cooking pot and place a trivet in the bottom. Place 2 custard cups on the trivet and place a second trivet on top. Place the remaining 2 cups on it. Lock lid in place. Select High Pressure and 6 minutes cook time.

When the cook time ends, turn off the instant cooker. Let the pressure release naturally for 5 minutes and finish with a quick pressure release. When the valve drops, carefully open the lid and remove the cups.

Nutrition Facts

Calories162, Total Fat 10.1g, Saturated Fat 3.6g, Cholesterol 331mg , Sodium 499mg, Total Carbohydrate 5.4g, Dietary Fiber 0.9g, Total Sugars 2.5g, Protein 13.1g

Peanut Butter and Mocha Smoothie

Preparation time: 5 minutes Cooking time: 0 minute

Servings: 1

Ingredients:

1 frozen banana, chopped

1 scoop of chocolate protein powder

2 tablespoons rolled oats

1/8 teaspoon sea salt

¼ teaspoon vanilla extract, unsweetened

1 teaspoon cocoa powder, unsweetened

2 tablespoons peanut butter

1 shot of espresso

½ cup almond milk, unsweetened

Directions:

Place all the ingredients in the order in a food processor or blender and then pulse for 2 to 3 minutes at high speed until smooth. Pour the smoothie into a glass and then serve.

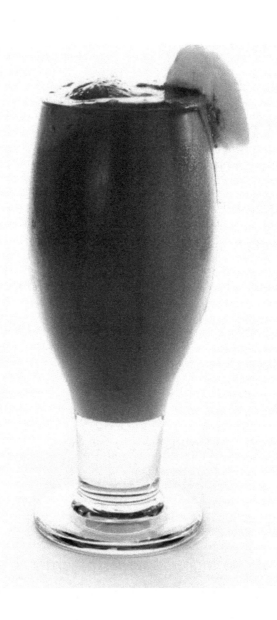

Sweet Potato Smoothie

Preparation time: 5 minutes Cooking time: 0 minute

Servings: 1

Ingredients:

1/2 cup frozen zucchini pieces

1 cup cubed cooked sweet potato, frozen

1/2 frozen banana

1/2 teaspoon sea salt

1/2 teaspoon cinnamon

1 scoop of vanilla protein powder

1/4 teaspoon nutmeg

1 tablespoon almond butter

1 1/2 cups almond milk, unsweetened

Directions:

Place all the ingredients in the order in a food processor or blender and then pulse for 2 to 3 minutes at high speed until smooth. Put the smoothie into a glass and then serve.

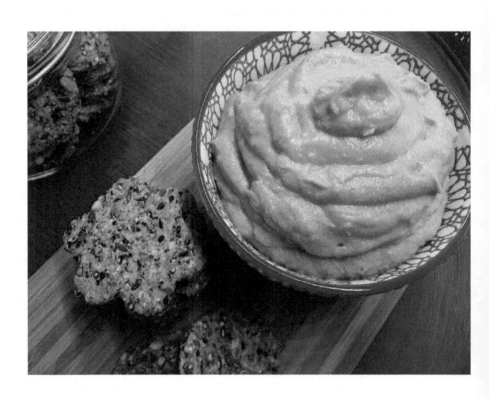

Lemon and Blueberry Smoothie

Preparation time: 5 minutes Cooking time: 0 minute

Servings: 1

Ingredients:

1 1/2 cups frozen blueberries

1/2 frozen banana

1 tablespoon chia seeds

3 tablespoon lemon juice

1 teaspoon lemon zest 1 1/2 teaspoon cinnamon

1 1/2 cups almond milk, unsweetened

1 scoop of vanilla protein powder

Directions:

Blend all the ingredients for 2 to 3 minutes at high speed until smooth. Pour the smoothie into a glass and then serve.

Beet and Orange Smoothie

Preparation time: 5 minutes Cooking time: 0 minute

Servings: 1

Ingredients:

1 cup chopped zucchini rounds, frozen

1 cup spinach

1 small peeled navel orange, frozen

1 small chopped beet

1 scoop of vanilla protein powder

1 cup almond milk, unsweetened

Directions:

Place all the ingredients in the order in a food processor or blender and then pulse for 2 to 3 minutes at high speed until smooth. Pour the smoothie into a glass and then serve

Chocolate, Avocado, and Banana Smoothie

Preparation time: 5 minutes Cooking time: 0 minute

Servings: 1

Ingredients:

1 medium frozen banana

2 small dates, pitted

1/2 cup steamed and frozen cauliflower florets

1/4 of a medium avocado

1 teaspoon cinnamon

1 tablespoon cacao powder

1/2 teaspoon sea salt

1 teaspoon maca

1/2 scoop of vanilla protein powder

2 tablespoon cacao nibs

1 tablespoon almond butter

1 cup almond milk

Directions:

Place all the ingredients in the order in a food processor or blender and then pulse for 2 to 3 minutes at high speed until smooth. Pour the smoothie into a glass and then serve.

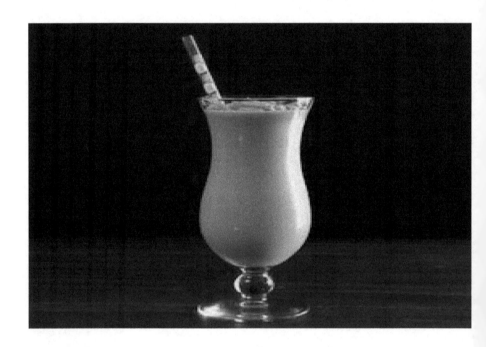

Scrambled Tofu Breakfast Tacos

Preparation time: 6 minutes Cooking time: 10 minutes
Servings: 4

Ingredients:

12 ounces tofu, pressed, drained

1/2 cup grape tomatoes, quartered

1 medium red pepper, diced

1 medium avocado, sliced

1 clove of garlic, minced

1/4 teaspoon ground turmeric

1/4 teaspoon ground black pepper

1/4 teaspoon salt

1/4 teaspoon cumin

1 teaspoon olive oil

8 corn tortillas

Directions:

Take a skillet pan, place it over medium heat, add oil and when hot, add pepper and garlic and cook for 2 minutes.

Then add tofu, crumble it, sprinkle with black pepper, salt, and all the spices, stir and cook for 5 minutes. When done, distribute tofu between tortilla, top with tomato and avocado, and serve.

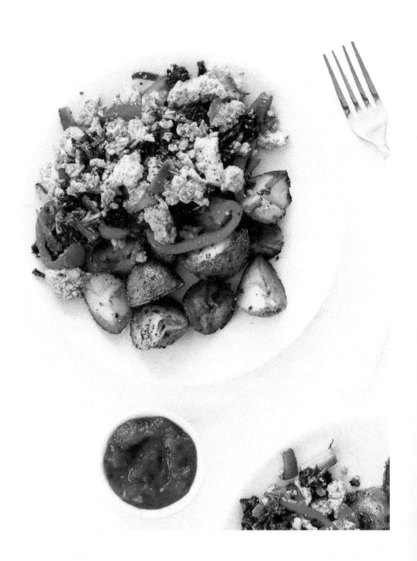

Lunch
Eggplant Curry

Prep time: 15 min Cooking Time: 15 min Serve: 2

Ingredients

1 large eggplant, peeled and chopped

½ cup green peas

½ cup cauliflowers

½ cup diced tomatoes

1 small onion, diced

1 teaspoon garlic, minced

¼ tablespoon curry powder

½ teaspoon Garam masala

½ teaspoon chili powder

½ teaspoon salt

½ teaspoon ground black pepper

Instructions

Add eggplants, green peas, cauliflowers, tomatoes, onions, minced garlic, curry powder, Garam masala, chili powder, salt, and pepper; mix well in an Instant Pot.

Secure the lid on the pot. Close the pressure-release valve. Select Manual and set the pot at High Pressure for 5 minutes. At the end of the cooking time, allow the pot to sit undisturbed for 10 minutes, then release any remaining.

Nutrition Facts

Calories 102, Total Fat 0.8g, Saturated Fat 0g, Cholesterol 0mg, Sodium 591mg, Total Carbohydrate 20.3g, Dietary Fiber 10.1g, Total Sugars 9.6g, Protein 3.4g

Potato, Apple, and Blueberries

Prep time: 15 min Cooking Time: 15 min Serve: 2

Ingredients

2 large potatoes, peeled and cut into 1-inch cubes

½ large apple, peeled and diced

½ cup blueberries

1/3 cup orange juice

¼ cup maple syrup

¼ teaspoon ground cinnamon

1/8 teaspoon ground nutmeg

1/8 teaspoon salt

½ tablespoon melted butter

1/2 cup toasted, chopped walnuts

Instructions

Select Sauté on the Instant Pot. When the pot is hot, add butter once the butter is melted. Combine potatoes, apple, blueberries, orange juice, maple syrup, ground cinnamon, ground nutmeg, walnuts, and salt.

Secure the lid on the Instant Pot. Close the pressure-release valve. Select Manual and set the pot at High Pressure for 5 minutes. At the end of the cooking time, allow the pot to sit undisturbed for 10 minutes, then release any remaining.

Nutrition Facts

Calories 518, Total Fat 8.3g, Saturated Fat 2.4g, Cholesterol 8mg, Sodium 195mg, Total Carbohydrate 102.9g, Dietary Fiber 11.8g, Total Sugars 40.8g, Protein 8g

Sweet Potato Beans and Cauliflower Curry

Prep time: 10 min Cooking Time: 10 min Serve: 2

Ingredients

1 onion, chopped

1 yellow bell peppers, seeded and chopped

1 teaspoon garlic powder

1 teaspoon ginger powder

½ teaspoon cumin seeds

¼ teaspoon salt

¼ teaspoon coriander powder

¼ teaspoon cinnamon powder

1/8 teaspoon red chili powder

2 cups water

2 sweet potatoes, peeled and chopped into 2-inch pieces

1 cup diced tomatoes

1/4 cup butter

1 cup sliced green beans

½ cup cauliflower, diced

Instructions

Place onion, yellow bell pepper, garlic powder, ginger powder, cumin seeds, salt, coriander powder, cinnamon powder, and chili powder in an Instant Pot. Pour in water and stir to combine. Mix in sweet potatoes, tomatoes, cauliflower, green beans, and butter.

Secure the lid on the pot. Close the pressure-release valve. Select Manual and set the pot at High Pressure for 5 minutes. At the end of the cooking time, allow the pot to sit undisturbed for 10 minutes, then release any remaining.

Serve hot.

Nutrition Facts

Calories 490, Total Fat 24g, Saturated Fat 14.7g, Cholesterol 61mg, Sodium 495mg, Total Carbohydrate 62.1g, Dietary Fiber 12g, Total Sugars 10.2g, Protein 6.5g

Corn Chowder

Prep time: 10 min Cooking Time: 15 min Serve: 2

Ingredients

1 cup sweet corn

½ cup potatoes, diced

1 tablespoon butter

1 small red onion, chopped

1red bell peppers, chopped

1 stalk leek, chopped

1 carrot, chopped

1 zucchini, chopped

½ cup broccoli, chopped

Salt and pepper to taste

½ cup coconut cream

2 cups water

Instructions

Select Sauté on the Instant Pot. When the pot is hot, add butter. Once the butter is melted, cook and stir red onion, corn, potatoes, red bell peppers, leeks, carrots, zucchinis, broccoli, salt, and pepper in the melted butter until onions are slightly translucent for 10-15 minutes. Stir vegetable mixture, add water.

Secure the lid on the pot. Close the pressure-release valve. Select Manual and set the pot at High Pressure for 15 minutes. At the end of the cooking time, allow the pot to sit undisturbed for 10 minutes, then release any remaining.

Open the lid and mix coconut cream.

Serve.

Nutrition Facts

Calories 271, Total Fat 7.3g, Saturated Fat 3.9g, Cholesterol 15mg, Sodium 104mg, Total Carbohydrate 44.2g, Dietary Fiber 7.6g, Total Sugars 12.6g, Protein 7g

Millet Pilaf with Mushrooms

Prep time: 10 min Cooking Time: 20 min serve: 2

Ingredients

1 tablespoon avocado oil

¼ teaspoon garlic powder

1 cup fresh shiitake mushroom caps, thinly sliced

1/8 teaspoon fine sea salt

1 1/2 cups vegetable broth

½ cup millet

1 small onion

½ cup green peas

1 carrot, chopped

Freshly ground black pepper

Salt to taste

1 tablespoon chopped cilantro

Instructions

Select the Sauté setting on the Instant Pot, add the avocado oil and garlic powder, and heat for 2 minutes until the garlic is bubbling. Add the mushrooms and salt and sauté for 3 minutes until the mushrooms are wilted. Stir in the broth. Stir in the millet, onions, carrots, green peas, and pepper, making sure all of the millet is fully submerged in the broth.

Secure the lid and set the Pressure Release to Sealing. Press the Cancel button to reset the cooking program. Then select the Manual or Pressure Cook setting and set the cooking time for 15 minutes at High Pressure. When the cooking program ends, let the pressure release naturally for 10 minutes, then move the pressure release to Vent to release any remaining steam. Open the pot and use a fork to fluff the buckwheat. Spoon onto plates, garnish with cilantro, and serve warm.

Nutrition Facts

Calories 262, Total Fat 3.9g, Saturated Fat 0.8g, Cholesterol 0mg, Sodium 582mg, Total Carbohydrate 48.7g, Dietary Fiber 6.3g, Total Sugars 3.4g, Protein 9.3g

Broccoli and Rice Stir Fry

Prep time: 5 min Cooking Time: 15 min serve: 2

Ingredients

½ cup uncooked long-grain rice

½ tablespoon coconut oil

½ cup broccoli florets, thawed

1 leek, diced

1 egg, beaten

1 cup vegetable broth

½ tablespoon soy sauce

1/8 teaspoon salt

1/8 teaspoon ground black pepper

Instructions

Press Sauté; heat coconut oil in Instant Pot.

Sauté broccoli until tender-crisp, and add leek.

Add egg, rice, broth, soy sauce, salt, and pepper.

Secure lid and move pressure release valve to Sealing. Press Manual or Pressure Cook; cook at High Pressure 6 minutes.

When cooking is complete, press Cancel and use Quick Release.

Serve hot.

Nutrition Facts

Calories 267, Total Fat 6.1g, Saturated

Fat 3.7g, Cholesterol 82mg, Sodium 422mg,

Total Carbohydrate

45.3g, Dietary Fiber 2.1g, Total Sugars 2.4g,

Protein 7.6g

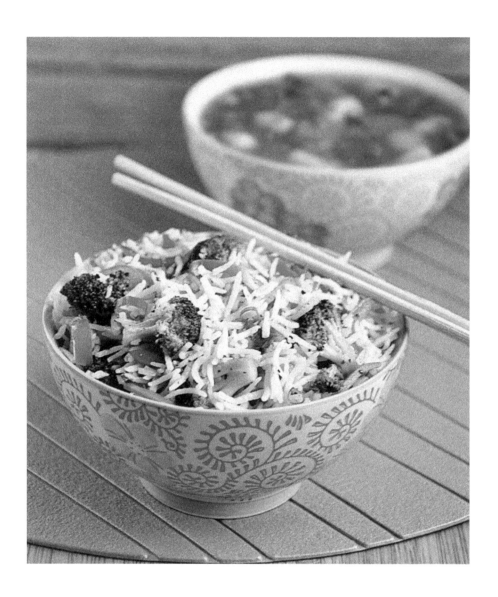

Tomato, Broccoli, and mint with Rice

Prep time: 5 min Cooking Time: 15 min serve: 2

Ingredients

1 1/2 cups water

1 cup milk

1 tablespoon butter

½ cup minced onion

½ teaspoon garlic powder

1 cup uncooked basmati rice

½ medium tomato, peeled, seeded, and chopped

½ cup fresh broccoli

1/2 cup grated parmesan cheese

1/2 cup fresh mint leaves, cut into thin strips

¼ teaspoon salt

Ground black pepper to taste

Instructions

Add butter to the Instant Pot. Using the display panel select the Sauté function and adjust to More or High.

When butter is melted, add sliced broccoli, tomato. Cook, occasionally stirring for 7 minutes, then

drain off any excess liquid. Add water and milk and stir. Turn the Instant Pot off by selecting Cancel, then secure the lid, making sure the vent is closed. Using the display panel, select the Manual or Pressure Cook function. Use the + /- keys and program

the Instant Pot for 6 minutes. When the time is up, quickly release the remaining pressure. Stir in parmesan cheese until melted. Adjust seasonings as needed.

Serve immediately garnished with chopped mint.

Nutrition Facts

Calories 514, Total Fat 10.6g, Saturated Fat 6.3g, Cholesterol 30mg, Sodium 481mg, Total Carbohydrate 89.7g, Dietary Fiber 5.8g, Total Sugars 8.1g, Protein 14.7g

Brown Rice, Cauliflower, Goat Cheese and Pecans Surprise

Prep time: 15 min Cooking Time: 20 min serve: 2

Ingredients

¼ cup chopped pecans

½ tablespoon butter

1 small onion, chopped

½ teaspoon garlic powder

½ cup uncooked brown rice

½ cup vegetable broth

½ fresh cauliflower florets

½ teaspoon salt

⅛ teaspoon ground black pepper

¼ cup shredded goat cheese

Instructions

Melt butter in an Instant Pot. Cook onions and garlic powder in melted butter for 3 minutes, stirring frequently. Stir in the cauliflower, brown rice, broth, salt, and pepper. Cover the lid. Using the display panel, select the Manual or Pressure Cook function. Use the + /- keys and program the Instant Pot for 6 minutes.

When the time is up, quickly release the remaining pressure.

Sprinkle pecans and cheese on top.

Nutrition Facts

Calories 287, Total Fat 7.2g, Saturated Fat 3.2g, Cholesterol 11mg, Sodium 851mg, Total Carbohydrate

48.1g, Dietary Fiber 6.2g, Total Sugars 5.4g, Protein 9.4g

Mexican Rice

Prep time: 15 min Cooking Time: 20 min serve: 2

Ingredients

½ teaspoons coconut oil

1/2 small onion, diced

½ cup uncooked long-grain rice

¼ teaspoon cumin seed

1/8 teaspoon chili powder

1 cup diced tomatoes

¼ teaspoon salt

1 cup water

Instructions

Select Sauté, and pour in the coconut oil. Once hot. Add the onions, cumin seed, and sauté for 3 to 4 minutes until the onion is translucent. Mix in the tomatoes, chili powder, and salt. Add the rice and water, and mix again.

Lock the lid into place. Select Pressure Cook or Manual, and adjust the pressure to High and the time to 3 minutes. Make sure the vent is set to

—Sealing‖.

After cooking, naturally, release the pressure for 3 minutes, then quickly release any remaining pressure. Unlock and remove the lid. Let the rice cool for 15 minutes. Using a fork, fluff the rice.

Serve hot.

Nutrition Facts

Calories 203, Total Fat 1.7g, Saturated Fat 1.1g, Cholesterol 0mg, Sodium 304mg, Total Carbohydrate 42.3g, Dietary Fiber 2.1g, Total Sugars 3.2g, Protein 4.4g

Tofu Pulao

Prep time: 10 min Cooking Time:15min serve: 2

Ingredients

1 tablespoon coconut oil

1 teaspoon cumin seeds

1 onion, sliced

1 green chili, chopped (or to taste)

½ tablespoon ginger garlic paste

1 big tomato, chopped

1 cup basmati rice

2 cups tofu

Mint to garnish

2 cups water

½ teaspoon turmeric powder

1 tablespoon coriander powder

Salt to taste

2 teaspoons Garam masala

Mint for garnishing

Instructions

Press Sauté mode on High Pressure. Add coconut oil; when hot, add cumin seeds fry well.

Add onions and green chilies, fry till onions turn slightly golden. Add ginger-garlic paste and fry well for 2 minutes or so. Add tomatoes and fry for 3 minutes or until mushy. Add turmeric powder, coriander powder, red chili powder, salt, and Garam masala and mix well.

Add tofu and rice along with water and mix. Turn off Sauté mode. Cover with the lid of Instant Pot, make sure the vent is set to Sealing, and push the Rice button. 6. Do a natural release or quick release after 2 minutes in Warm mode. Garnish with mint.

Nutrition Facts

Calories 650, Total Fat 20.7g, Saturated Fat 3.3g, Cholesterol 0mg, Sodium 134mg, Total Carbohydrate

86.9g, Dietary Fiber 5.7g, Total Sugars 5.5g, Protein 29.2g

Soups and Salads

Mexican Spaghettini Soup

Ingredients

5 large tomatoes, cut into large cubes

1 medium red onion, cut into large cubes

3 cloves garlic

2 Tbsp. olive oil

16 oz. spaghettini, broken into 1-inch pieces

32 oz. vegetable broth

1/2 tsp. sea salt

1/2 Tbsp. black pepper

2 Tbsp. oregano

2 Tbsp. cumin Chili flakes, chopped Serrano chilies, or diced jalapeños, to taste (optional)

Directions:

Cilantro, sour soy cream, and sliced avocado for garnish (optional) Puree the tomatoes, red onions, garlic, and oil. Transfer to a and cook on medium heat. Add in the noodles, broth, salt, pepper, oregano, and cumin. Add the chili flakes, Serrano chilies. Cook for 13 ½ minutes and simmer until the noodles become tender. Garnish with cilantro, sour soy cream, or avocado.

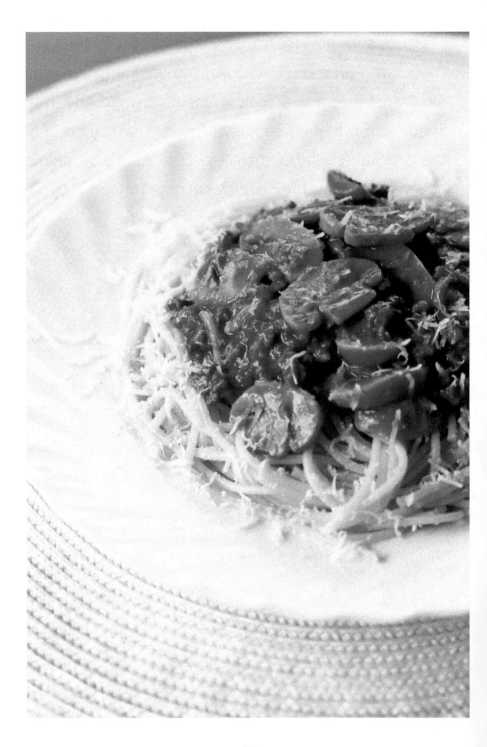

Split Pea Celery and Leek Soup

Ingredients

16- oz package

1 lb dried green split peas, rinsed

1 large leek light green and a white portion only, chopped and thoroughly cleaned

3 celery ribs diced

2 large carrots diced

4 garlic clove minced

1/4 cup chopped fresh parsley

6 cups vegetable broth

1/2 t ground black pepper

1 bay leaf

Directions:

Pour all of the ingredients into a slow cooker and combine thoroughly. Cover a cook on low heat for 7 and a half hours or high 3 and a half hours. Take out the bay leaf.

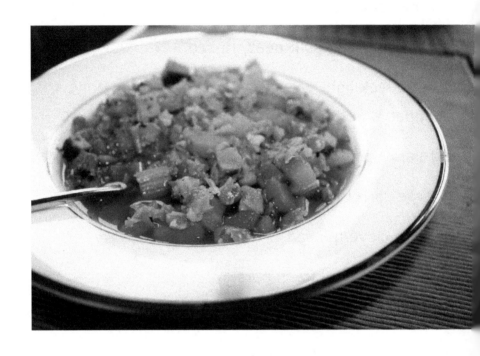

Red Potato and Baby Spinach Soup

Ingredients

5 cups low sodium vegetable stock

3 large red potatoes peeled and chopped

1 cup onion chopped

2 stalks celery chopped

4 cloves garlic crushed

1 cup heavy cream

1 tsp. dried tarragon

2 cups baby spinach 6-8 Tbsp. sliced almonds, sea salt, and ground black pepper to taste

Directions:

Combine stock, sweet potatoes, onion, celery, and garlic to a 4-quart slow cooker. Cook on low heat for 8 hours or until potatoes become soft. Add almond milk, tarragon, salt, and pepper. Blend this mixture for 1-2 minutes with an immersion blender until the soup is smooth. Add baby spinach & cover. Let it rest for 20 minutes or until spinach becomes soft. Garnish with almonds and season with sea salt and pepper.

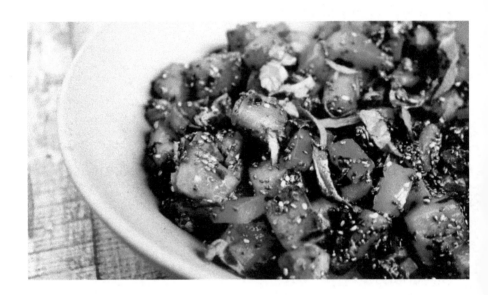

Garnish with lemon Slow Cooked Lima Bean Soup

Ingredients

1 Tbsp extra virgin olive oil

6 cloves garlic, minced

1 medium red onion, diced

1/2 lb carrots, sliced thinly into rounds

4 stalks celery (1/2 bunch), sliced

1 lb dry lima beans, stones removed, rinsed, and drained

1 whole bay leaf

1 tsp dried rosemary

1/2 tsp dried thyme

1/2 tsp Spanish paprika Freshly cracked pepper (15-20 cranks of a pepper mill)

1 1/2 tsp salt or more to taste

Directions:

Put the olive oil, garlic, onion, celery, and carrots into the slow cooker.

Add the beans, bay leaf, rosemary, thyme, paprika, and some freshly cracked pepper to the slow cooker.

Add 6 cups of water to the slow cooker and combine the ingredients. Cover and cook for 8 hours on low or on high for 4 1/2 hours.

Once it's cooked, stir the soup and mash the beans. Season with more sea salt, if necessary.

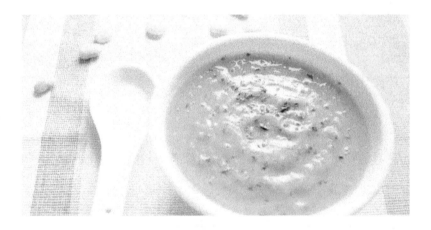

Carrot and Cardamom Soup

Ingredients

1 large red onion, finely chopped

4 fat garlic cloves, crushed

1 large carrot, finely chopped thumb-sized piece of ginger, peeled and finely chopped

2 tbsp olive oil Pinch of turmeric Seeds from 10 cardamom pods

1 tsp cumin, seeds, or ground

¼ pound soy beans

1 ¾ cup coconut milk zest and juice

1 lemon pinch of chili flakes handful of parsley, chopped

Directions:

Heat some oil in a pan and cook the onions, garlic, carrot, and ginger until softened. Add in the turmeric, cardamom, and cumin. Cook for a few mins more until the spices become aromatic. Add the soy beans, coconut milk, 1 cup of water. Boil and reduce to a simmer for 15 mins until the soy beans become soft. A process with a hand blender, pulse the soup until it's chunky. Garnish with lemon zest and juice. Season with salt, chili, and herbs. Divide among bowls and sprinkle with more lemon zest.

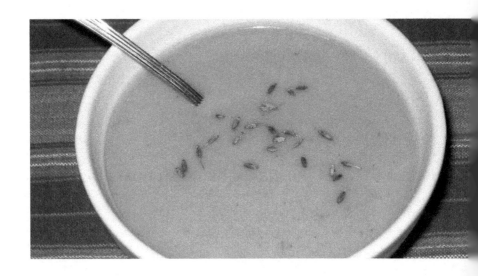

Lettuce Tomatillos and Almond Salad

Ingredients:

6 to 7 cups lettuce,

3 bundles, trimmed

1/4 cucumber, halved lengthwise, then thinly sliced

3 tablespoons chopped or snipped chives

16 tomatillos, sliced in half

1/2 cup sliced almonds

1/4 white onion, sliced Salt, and pepper, to taste

3 ounces cream cheese, crumbled

3 ounces Camembert cheese, crumbled

3 ounces mozzarella cheese, shredded

Dressing:

1 sprig cilantro, minced

1 tablespoon distilled white vinegar

1/4 lemon, juiced, about 2 teaspoons

1/4 cup extra-virgin olive oil

1 tsp. English mustard Prep

Directions:

Combine all of the dressing ingredients in a food processor. Toss with the rest of the ingredients and combine well.

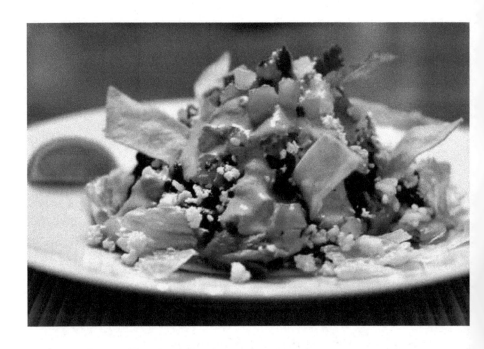

Kale Almond and Vegan Ricotta Salad

Ingredients:

6 to 7 cups kale,

3 bundles, trimmed

1/4 cucumber, halved lengthwise, then thinly sliced

3 tablespoons chopped or snipped chives

16 green tomatillos, sliced in half

1/2 cup sliced almonds

1/4 white onion, sliced Salt, and pepper, to taste

3 ounces cottage cheese, crumbled

3 ounces pepper jack cheese, shredded

3 ounces pecorino romano cheese, shredded

Dressing:

1 tablespoon distilled white vinegar

1/4 lemon, juiced, about

2 teaspoons

1/4 cup extra- virgin olive oil

1 tsp. Dijon mustard Prep Combine all of the dressing ingredients in a food processor.

Directions:

Toss with the rest of the ingredients and combine well.

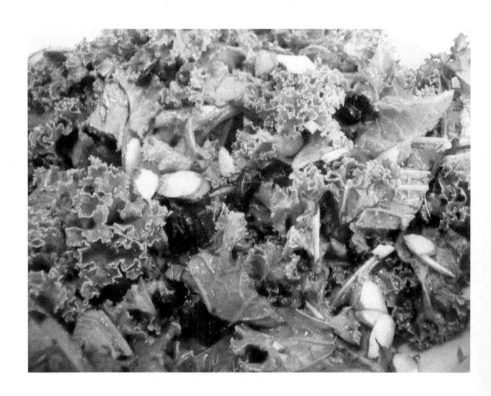

Mesclun Tomatillo and Almond Salad

Ingredients:

6 to 7 cups mesclun,

3 bundles, trimmed

1/4 cucumber, halved lengthwise, then thinly sliced

3 tablespoons chopped or snipped chives

16 tomatillos, sliced in half

1/2 cup sliced almonds

1/4 white onion, sliced Salt, and pepper, to taste

3 ounces feta cheese, crumbled

3 ounces ricotta cheese

3 ounces cheddar cheese, shredded

1 tablespoon distilled white vinegar

1/4 lemon, juiced, about

2 teaspoons

1/4 cup extra-virgin olive oil

1 tsp. egg-free mayonnaise Prep

Directions:

Combine all of the dressing ingredients in a food processor. Toss with the rest of the ingredients and combine well.

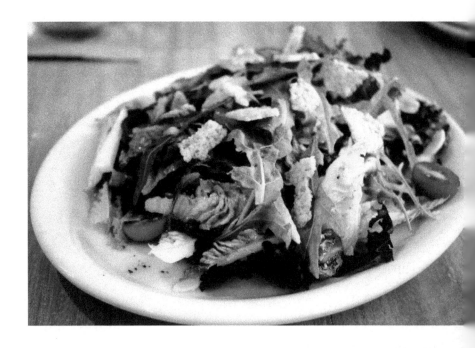

Bib Lettuce Tomatillo and Almond Salad

Ingredients:

6 to 7 cups bib lettuce,

3 bundles, trimmed

1/4 cucumber, halved lengthwise, then thinly sliced

3 tablespoons chopped or snipped chives

16 tomatillos, sliced in half

1/2 cup sliced almonds

1/4 white onion, sliced

Salt and pepper, to taste

3 ounces Monterey jack cheese, shredded

3 ounces feta cheese, crumbled

3 ounces ricotta cheese

Dressing:

1 tablespoon distilled white vinegar

1/4 lemon, juiced, about

2 teaspoons

1/4 cup extra-virgin olive oil

1 tsp. Dijon mustard Prep

Directions:

Combine all of the dressing ingredients in a food processor. Toss with the rest of the ingredients and combine well.

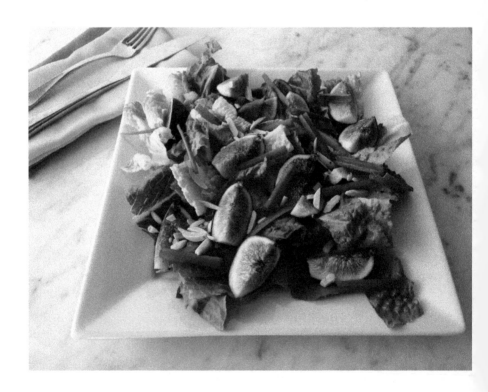

Butter Lettuce and Feta Cheese Salad

Ingredients:

6 to 7 cups butter lettuce,

3 bundles, trimmed

1/4 cucumber, halved lengthwise, then thinly sliced

3 tablespoons chopped or snipped chives

16 tomatillos, sliced in half

1/2 cup sliced almonds

1/4 white onion, sliced

Salt and pepper, to taste

6 ounces Monterey jack cheese, shredded

3 ounces feta cheese, crumbled

Dressing:

1 sprig cilantro, minced

1 tablespoon distilled white vinegar

1/4 lemon, juiced, about

2 teaspoons

1/4 cup extra-virgin olive oil

1 tsp. egg-free mayonnaise

Prep Combine all of the dressing ingredients in a food processor.

Directions:

Toss with the rest of the ingredients and combine well.

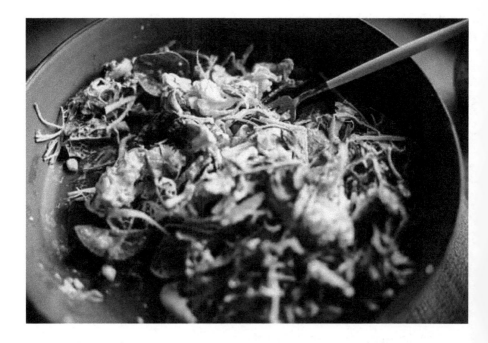

Dinner

Quick Spiralized Zucchini and Grape Tomatoes

Prep Time: 5 mins Cook Time: 10 mins Total Time: 15 mins Servings: 2 servings

Ingredients

1/2 tablespoon olive oil

3 garlic cloves, chopped

3/4 lb grape tomatoes, cut in half pinch red crushed pepper flakes

Kosher Salt and freshly ground black pepper, to taste

1 tbsp chopped fresh basil

1 large zucchini, spiralized with thicker blade

Instructions

In a large non-stick pan set over high heat, heat the oil. Add the garlic and cook until golden, 30 seconds.

Add the tomatoes, and crushed red pepper flakes, and season with salt and pepper. Reduce the heat to low.

Simmer, covered, until the tomatoes soften, 15 minutes. Increase heat to medium-high, stir in the zucchini and basil, season with salt and cook 2 minutes. Serve right away.

Nutrition Info

Calories: 117kcal Carbohydrates: 20g Protein: 4g

Fat: 5g Sodium: 31mg Fiber: 5g Sugar: 2g

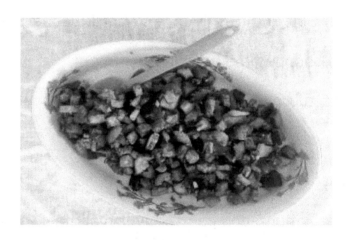

Tomato Basil and Mozzarella Galette

Servings: 3

Ingredients

1 cup almond flour 1 large egg

3 tablespoons mozzarella liquid 1 teaspoon garlic powder

¼ cup shredded Parmesan cheese 2 tablespoons pesto

3-4 leaves fresh basil

½ ounce Mozzarella pearls* 3-4 cherry tomatoes

Instructions

Heat oven to 375°F and line a cookie sheet with parchment. Spray with non stick spray. Combine the almond flour, garlic powder, and mozzarella liquid in a bowl then stir gently. Add the egg and Parmesan cheese then mix well until dough forms. Form the dough mixture into a large ball and place on the prepared parchment. Press the dough ball into a circle, working to keep the thickness uniform. It should press out to about ½ inch thick. It may be sticky so wetting your hands with a little water can help keep your fingers from picking up the crust. Spread pesto evenly over the center of the crust, leaving room to fold in the edges. Layer mozzarella, basil leaves, and tomatoes. Using the edge of the parchment, fold the edges of the crust up and over the filling. Work in a circle around the edge until all of the edges are folded up. Bake for 20 to 25 minutes or until crust browns and cheese is melted.

Nutrition Info

323.67 Calories

24.01 g Fat

7.87 g Net Carbs

14.46 g Protein.

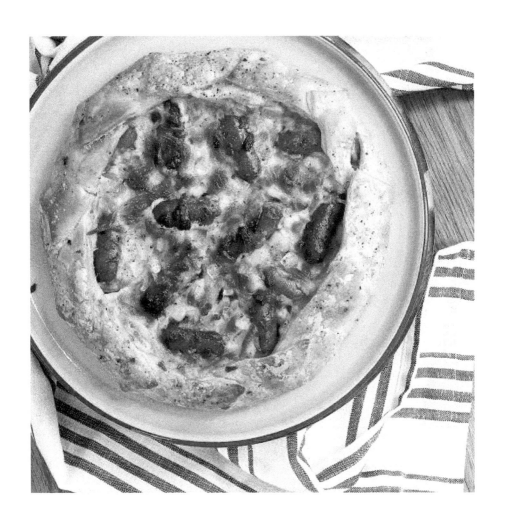

Zucchini Noodles with Avocado Sauce

Prep: 10 mins

Total: 10 mins

Servings 2

Ingredients

1 zucchini

1   1/4 cup basil (30 g) 1/3 cup water (85 ml) 4 tbsp pine nuts

2   tbsp lemon juice 1 avocado

12 sliced cherry tomatoes

Instructions

Make the zucchini noodles using a peeler or the Spiralizer. Blend the rest of the ingredients (except the cherry tomatoes) in a blender until smooth.

Combine noodles, avocado sauce and cherry tomatoes in a mixing bowl.

These zucchini noodles with avocado sauce are better fresh, but you can store them in the fridge for 1 to 2 days.

Notes

Feel free to use any veggies or fresh herbs you have on hand. You can also spiralize other veggies like carrots, beet, butternut squash, cabbage, etc.

Any nuts can be used instead of the pine nuts, or even seeds.

Nutrition Info

Serving Size: 1/2 of the recipe Calories: 313

Sugar: 6.5 g

Sodium: 22 mg

Fat: 26.8 g

Saturated Fat: 3.1 g Carbohydrates: 18.7 g

Fiber: 9.7 g

Protein: 6.8 g

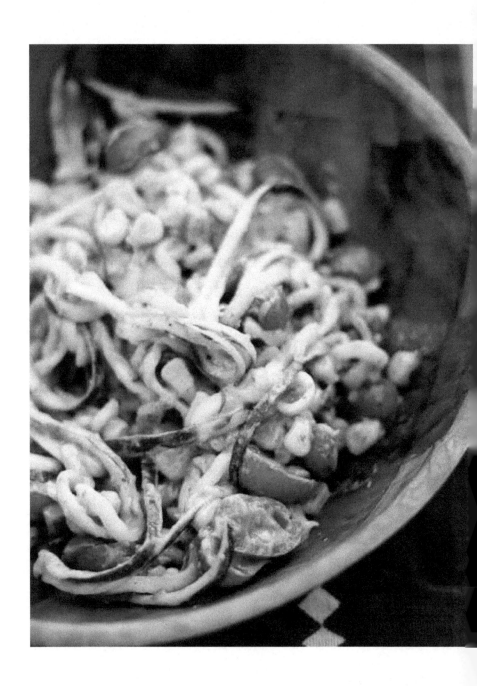

Cheesy Spaghetti Squash with Pesto

Servings: 4 servings

Ingredients

2 cups cooked spaghetti squash, drained

1 Tbsp olive oil

salt and pepper to taste

1/2 cup whole milk ricotta cheese

Instructions

In a medium-sized bowl combine the squash and olive oil. Season with salt and pepper to taste. Spread the squash about 2 inches deep in an oven proof casserole dish.

Drop ricotta cheese on top by the spoonful. Scatter the cubes of mozzarella cheese over the top. Bake for about 10 minutes in a 375 degree (F) oven, or until the cheese has melted and is bubbly.

Remove from the oven, cool for about 5 minutes, then drizzle the pesto over the top and serve.

Nutrition Info

207 calories 17g fat 4.8g net carbs 11g protein

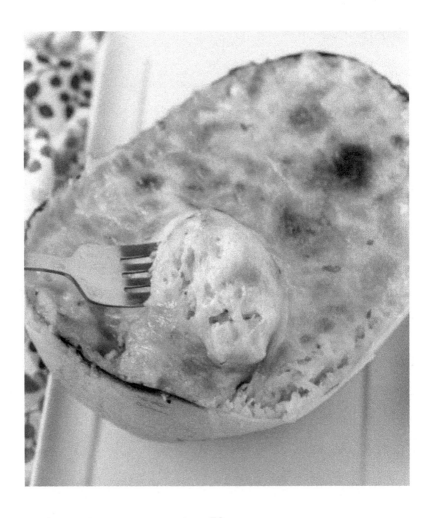

Easy Keto Broccoli Slaw Recipe

Servings: 6 servings

Ingredients

1 Tbsp extra virgin olive oil 1/3 cup sugar free mayonnaise 1 1/2 Tbsp apple cider vinegar 1 Tbsp dijon mustard

2   Tbsp granulated sugar substitute 1 tsp celery seeds

1/2 tsp kosher salt (or more to taste) 1/4 tsp black pepper

4 cups bagged broccoli slaw

Instructions

In a large bowl, whisk the olive oil, mayonnaise, apple cider vinegar, mustard, sugar substitute, celery seeds, salt and pepper together until fully combined. Add the broccoli slaw. Toss well to coat. Serve cold.

 Nutrition Info 110 calories 10g fat 2g net carbs 2g protein.

White Beans and Italian Sausage Burrito Bowl

Ingredients

1 red onion, diced or thinly sliced

1 green bell pepper (I used yellow), diced

1 mild red chili, finely chopped

1 1/2 cup white beans

1/2 cup vegan Italian sausage, crumbled

1 cup uncooked white rice

1 1/2 cups chopped tomatoes

1/2 cup water

4 tbsp. pesto

1 tsp. Italian seasoning

Sea salt Black pepper

Toppings: fresh coriander (cilantro), chopped spring onions, sliced avocado, guacamole, etc.

Directions:

Combine all the burrito bowl ingredients (not toppings) in a slow cooker. Cook on low for 3 hours, or until the rice is cooked. Serve hot with topping ingredients.

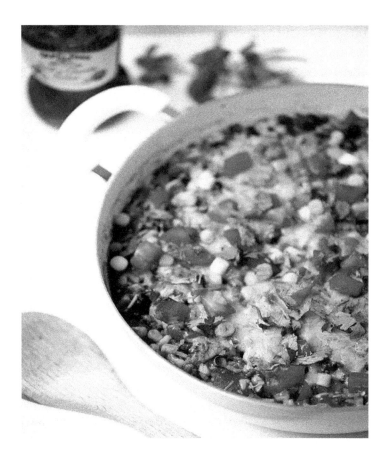

Smoky Red Rice with Garbanzo Beans

Ingredients

1 poblano chili, diced

1 red onion, diced

1 mild red chili, finely chopped

1/2 cup vegan burger (Brand: Beyond Meat Beyond Burger), crumbled

1 ½ cups garbanzo beans, drained

1 cup uncooked red rice

1 ½ cups chopped tomatoes

½ cup water

4 tbsp. chimichurri sauce

1/2 tsp. cayenne pepper

Sea salt Black pepper

Toppings: fresh coriander (cilantro), chopped spring onions, sliced avocado, guacamole, etc.

Directions:

Combine all the burrito bowl ingredients (not toppings) in a slow cooker. Cook on low for 3 hours, or until the rice is cooked. Serve hot with topping ingredients

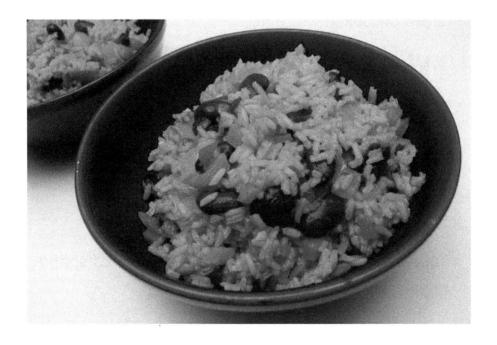

Vegan Chorizo Burrito Bowl

Ingredients

1 ancho chili, diced

1 red onion, diced

1 mild red chili, finely chopped

1/2 cup vegan Chorizo (Soyrizo), crumbled

1 cup uncooked white rice

1 1/2 cups chopped tomatoes

1/2 cup water

1/4 cup vegan chorizos, coarsely chopped

1 tsp. dried thyme

Sea salt Black pepper

Toppings: fresh coriander (cilantro), chopped spring onions, sliced avocado, guacamole, etc.

Directions:

Combine all the burrito bowl ingredients (not toppings) in a slow cooker. Cook on low for 3 hours, or until the rice is cooked. Serve hot with topping ingredients

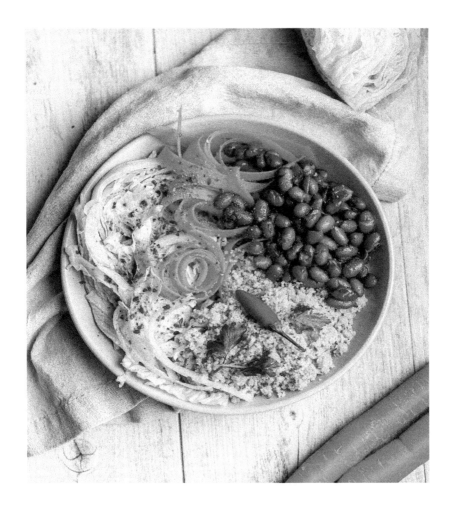

Chimichurri Vegan Chorizo Burrito Bowl

Ingredients

1 Anaheim pepper, diced

1 red onion, diced

1 mild red chili, finely chopped

1/2 cup vegan Chorizo (Soyrizo), crumbled

1 cup uncooked red rice

1 ½ cups chopped tomatoes

½ cup water

4 tbsp. chimichurri sauce

1/2 tsp. cayenne pepper

Sea salt Black pepper

Toppings: fresh coriander (cilantro), chopped spring onions, sliced avocado, guacamole, etc.

Directions:

Combine all the burrito bowl ingredients (not toppings) in a slow cooker. Cook on low for 3 hours, or until the rice is cooked. Serve hot with topping ingredients

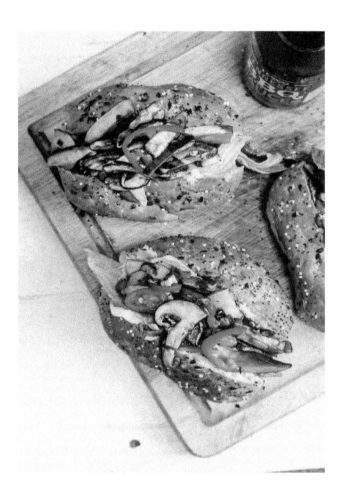

Smoky White Bean & White Rice Burrito Bowl

Ingredients

1 red onion, diced or thinly sliced

1/2 cup meatless meatballs, crumbled

1 mild red chili, finely chopped

1 1/2 cup white beans

1 cup uncooked white rice

1 1/2 cups chopped tomatoes

1/2 cup water

1 tbsp chipotle hot sauce (or other favorite hot sauce)

1 tsp smoked paprika

1/2 tsp ground cumin

Sea salt Black pepper

Toppings: fresh coriander (cilantro), chopped spring onions, sliced avocado, guacamole, etc.

Directions:

Combine all the burrito bowl ingredients (not toppings) in a slow cooker. Cook on low for 3 hours, or until the rice is cooked. Serve hot with topping ingredients

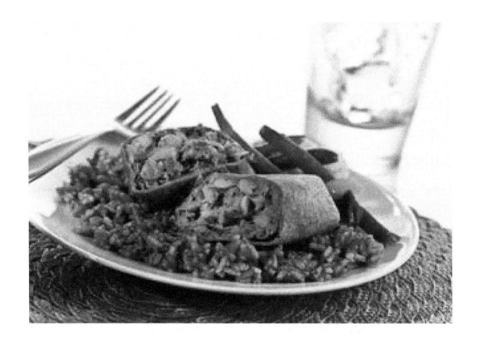

Sweets

Pecan Pie Muffins

Prep time: 15 min Cooking Time: 25 min serve: 2

Ingredients

1 tablespoon honey

1 cup coconut flour

1 tablespoon chopped pecans

1tablespoon butter, softened

1 egg, beaten

1 cup water

Instructions

In a medium bowl, stir together honey, coconut flour and pecans. In a separate bowl beat the butter and egg together until smooth, stir into the dry ingredients until combined. Spoon the batter into the prepared muffin cups.

Pour 1 cup water into the Instant Pot. Place the trivet inside. Place the muffin cups on the rack or pan.

Secure the lid and set the Pressure Release valve to Sealing. Press the Pressure Cook or Manual button and set the cook time to 25 minutes.

When the Instant Pot beeps, allow the pressure to release naturally for 10 minutes, then carefully switch the

Pressure Release valve to Venting. When fully released, open the lid. Carefully remove the muffins.

Nutrition Facts

Calories 97, Total Fat 7g, Saturated Fat 2.9g, Cholesterol 49mg, Sodium 44mg, Total Carbohydrate

6.9g, Dietary Fiber 1.6g , Total Sugars 4.8g, Protein 2.3g

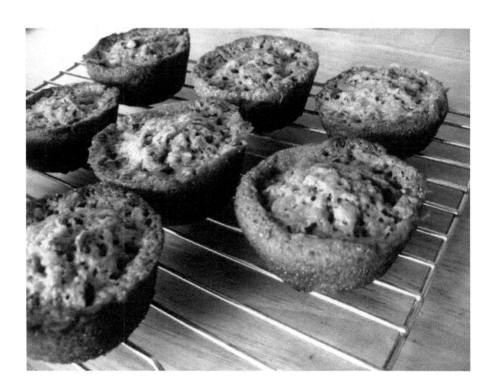

Spinach-Egg Muffins

Prep time: 10 min Cooking Time: 25 min serve: 2

Ingredients

1 cup spinach, chopped

2 eggs

¼ teaspoon salt

¼ teaspoon freshly ground black pepper

¼ teaspoon coconut oil

½ large white onion, chopped

1 cup water

Instructions

In a large bowl, whisk the eggs together and add the salt and pepper. Set aside.

In a pan, heat the coconut oil and sauté the onion until translucent for 3-5 minutes. Remove from the heat. Add the onion and spinach to the eggs and mix well.

Pour 1 cup water into the Instant Pot. Place the trivet inside. Place the muffin cups on the rack or pan.

Secure the lid and set the Pressure Release valve to Sealing. Press the Pressure Cook or Manual button and set the cook time to 20 minutes.

When the Instant Pot beeps, allow the pressure to release naturally for 10 minutes, then carefully switch the Pressure Release valve to Venting. When fully released, open the lid. Carefully remove the muffins.

Nutrition Facts

Calories 125, Total Fat 5.8g, Saturated Fat 2g, Cholesterol 164mg, Sodium 446mg, Total Carbohydrate 8.4g, Dietary Fiber 4.3g , Total Sugars 2.4g, Protein 9.8g

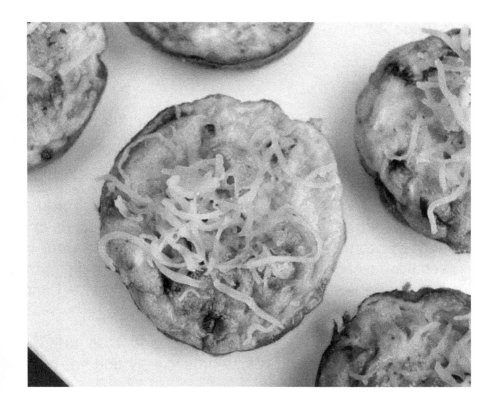

Crispy Tofu

Prep time: 5 min Cooking Time: 15 min serve: 2

Ingredients

1 cup tofu, cut into pieces for your choice

Salt and freshly-cracked black pepper

1 tablespoon butter

½ cup tomato sauce

½ tablespoon lime juice

Chopped fresh cilantro

Instructions

In a medium mixing bowl, whisk together the tomato sauce, lime juice combined. Set aside until ready to use

Season tofu pieces on all sides with salt and pepper.

Click the —Sauté‖ setting on theInstant Pot . Add the butter, followed tofu, turning every 45-60 seconds or so until the tofu is browned on all sides. Transfer tofu to a separate clean plate, and repeat with the remaining tofu searing until it has browned on all sides. Press —Cancel to turn off the heat.

Pour in the tomato sauce mixer, and toss briefly to combine with the tofu. Close lid securely and set vent to —Sealing

Cook on high pressure for 2 minutes, followed by natural release (about 15 minutes).

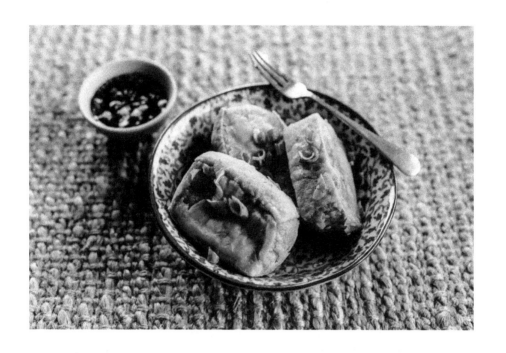

Plum Skillet Cake

Prep time: 15 min Cooking Time: 50 min serve: 2

Ingredients

2½ tablespoon coconut oil

½ cup almond flour

¼ teaspoon salt

¼ teaspoon baking powder

1/8 teaspoon baking soda

2 tablespoon honey

1 large egg

½ cup low-fat buttermilk

2 medium ripe plums, pitted and thinly sliced

2 tablespoons coconut sugar

Instructions

Butter an 8-inch cast iron or oven-proof skillet. Dust with flour, tapping out any excess.

Whisk together almond flour, salt, baking powder, and baking soda in a medium bowl.

Combine coconut oil and honey in a large bowl; beat with an electric mixer on medium speed until pale and fluffy. Beat in egg. Add flour mixture in 3 batches, alternating with buttermilk, beating batter briefly after each addition.

Pour batter into the prepared skillet and smooth the top with an offset spatula. Fan plum slices on top of batter, and sprinkle with remaining coconut sugar.

Pour 1 cup water into the Instant Pot and arrange the handled trivet on the bottom. Place the pan on top of the trivet and cover it with an upside-down plate or another piece of parchment to protect the brownies from condensation.

Secure the lid and move the steam release valve to Sealing. Select Manual/Pressure Cook to cook on high pressure for 45 minutes. When the cooking cycle is complete, let the pressure naturally release for 10 minutes, then move the steam release valve to Venting to release any remaining pressure. When the floating valve drops, remove the lid.

Let cool slightly before serving.

Nutrition Facts

Calories 396, Total Fat 37.3g, Saturated Fat 31.4g, Cholesterol 48mg, Sodium 236mg, Total Carbohydrate 14.4g, Dietary Fiber 0.5g, Total Sugars 13.7g, Protein 2.9g

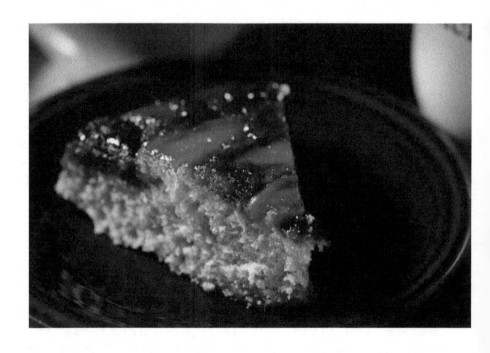

Yellow Squash Brownies

Prep time: 15 min Cooking Time: 45 min serve: 2

Ingredients

1 tablespoons coconut oil

½ tablespoons honey

½ teaspoon vanilla extract

1 cup coconut flour

½ tablespoon unsweetened cocoa powder

½ teaspoon baking soda

1/8 teaspoon salt

1 cup shredded yellow squash

¼ cup chopped walnuts

Instructions

Grease and flour a 9x13-inch baking pan.

In a large bowl, mix the coconut oil, honey and 2 teaspoons vanilla until well blended. Combine the coconut flour, cocoa, baking soda and salt; stir into the honey mixture. Fold in the yellow squash and walnuts. Spread evenly into the prepared pan.

Pour 1 cup water into the Instant Pot and arrange the handled trivet on the bottom. Place the pan on top of the trivet and cover it with an upside-down plate or another piece of parchment to protect the brownies from condensation.

Secure the lid and move the steam release valve to Sealing. Select Manual/Pressure Cook to cook on high pressure for 45 minutes. When the cooking cycle is complete, let the pressure naturally release for 10 minutes, then move the steam release valve to Venting to release any remaining pressure. When the floating valve drops, remove the lid.

Let cool slightly before serving.

Nutrition Facts

Calories 108, Total Fat 8.7g, Saturated Fat 3.8g, Cholesterol 0mg , Sodium 243mg, Total Carbohydrate

6.3g, Dietary Fiber 2.3g, Total Sugars 3.1g, Protein 2.9g

Winter wonderland cake

Prep:1 hr Cook:35 mins Plus cooling easy Serves 12
Ingredients

175g unsalted butter, softened, plus more for the tin
250g golden caster sugar

3 large eggs

225g plain flour

2 tsp baking powder 50g crème fraîche

100g dark chocolate, melted and cooled a little

3 tbsp strawberry jam

8-10 candy canes, red and white mini white meringues
and jelly sweets, to decorate

For the angel frosting

500g white caster sugar

1 tsp vanilla extract 1 tbsp liquid glucose

2 egg whites 30g icing sugar, sifted

Directions:

Heat oven to 180C/160C fan/gas 4. Butter and line three
18cm (or two 20cm) cake tins. Beat the butter and sugar
together until light and fluffy. Add the eggs, beating them
in one at a time. Fold in the flour, baking powder and a
pinch of salt, fold in the crème fraîche and chocolate and
100ml boiling water. 2 Divide the cake mixture between
the tins and level the tops the batter. Bake for 25-30
mins or until a skewer inserted into the middle comes out

clean. Leave to cool for 10 mins in the tin, then tip out onto a cooling rack and peel off the parchment. Set aside to cool completely. 3 To make the angel frosting, put the sugar, vanilla and liquid glucose in a pan with 125ml water. Bring to the boil and cook until the sugar has melted – the syrup turns transparent and the mixture hits 130C on a sugar thermometer (be very careful with hot sugar). Take off the heat.

Meanwhile, beat the egg whites until stiff then, while still beating, gradually pour in the hot sugar syrup in a steady stream. Keep beating until the mixture is fluffy and thick enough to spread – this might take a few mins as the mixture cools. Beat in the icing sugar. 4 Spread two of the sponges with jam and some of the icing mixture, then sandwich the cakes together with the plain one on top. Use a little of the frosting to ice the whole cake (don't worry about crumbs at this stage). Use the remaining icing to ice the cake again, smoothing the side, and swirling it on top. Crush four of the candy canes and sprinkle over the cake, then add the remaining whole candy canes, meringues and sweets.

Nutty cinnamon & yogurt dipper

Prep:5 mins No cook easy Serves 1

Ingredients

100g natural Greek yogurt

1 tbsp nut butter (try almond or cashew)

¼ tsp ground cinnamon 1 tsp honey To serve

apple wedges (tossed in a little lemon juice to prevent them turning brown)

celery sticks

carrot sticks

mini rice cakes or crackers (choose gluten-free brands if necessary)

Directions:

1 In a small tub, mix the yogurt, nut butter, cinnamon and honey. Serve with apple wedges (tossed in a little lemon juice to prevent them turning brown), celery or carrot sticks, and mini rice cakes or crackers.

Coconut bauble truffles

Prep:45 mins plus at least 2 hrs chilling, no cook Easy
Makes about 25

Ingredients

250g madeira cake

85g ready-to-eat dried apricots, finely chopped

25g desiccated coconut

125ml light condensed milk To decorate

140g desiccated coconut

different food colourings, we used yellow, pink, blue and
purple

Directions:

In a big mixing bowl, crumble the cake with your fingers
– try to get the bits as small as possible.

Tip in the apricots and coconut. Using your hands again,
mix with the cake crumbs. Use a wooden spoon to stir in
the condensed milk. After you've mixed it in a bit, use
your fingers to pull off any bits stuck to the spoon.
Squidge everything together with your hands until it is
well mixed and all the cake crumbs are sticky. Rub your
hands together over the bowl so any bits that are stuck
drop off.

Line some trays that fit in your fridge with baking
parchment. Roll the sticky cake mixture into small balls
(about the size of a conker or gobstopper) between your

hands. Line them up on the trays, then put them in the fridge while you get the decorations ready.

Decide how many different food colorings you will use, then split the coconut into the same number of piles. Put each pile of coconut into a plastic sandwich bag, add a few drops of food colouring to each, and tie a knot in the top. Shake the bags and scrunch between your fingers until all the coconut is coloured – if it's not bright enough, open the bag and add a few more drops of colouring.

Open all the bags of coloured coconut and take the truffles from the fridge. Put 1 tbsp of water in a small bowl and lightly coat each truffle in it so the coconut can stick to the outside of each bauble.

One by one, drop each truffle into one of your bags. Shake it and roll it around until the outside is covered in coconut. Carefully put each truffle back onto the trays and chill for at least another 2 hrs until they are freezing.

If you like, put some of the truffles in gift bags or boxes and tie with ribbons to give as presents. Will keep in the fridge for up to 1 week.

Christmas cake cupcakes

Prep:40 mins Cook:45 mins easy Makes 12

Ingredients

For the batter

200g dark muscovado sugar

175g butter

700g luxury mixed dried fruit

50g glacé cherries

2 tsp grated fresh root ginger zest and juice

1 orange

100ml dark rum, brandy or orange juice

85g/3oz pecan nuts, roughly chopped

3 large eggs, beaten

85g ground almond

200g plain flour ½ tsp baking powder

1 tsp mixed spice

1 tsp cinnamon For the icing

400g pack ready-rolled marzipan (we used Dr Oetker)

4 tbsp warm apricot jam or shredless marmalade

500g pack fondant icing sugar

icing sugar, for dusting

6 gold and 6 silver muffin cases 6 gold and 6 silver sugared almond

snowflake sprinkles

Directions:

Tip the sugar, butter, dried fruit, whole cherries, ginger, orange zest and juice into a large pan. Pour over the rum, brandy or juice, then put on the heat and slowly bring to the boil, stirring frequently to melt the butter. Reduce the heat and bubble gently, uncovered for 10 mins, stirring now and again to make sure the mixture doesn't catch on the bottom of the pan. Set aside for 30 mins to cool.

Stir the nuts, eggs and ground almonds into the fruit, then sift in the flour, baking powder and spices. Stir everything together gently but thoroughly. Your batter is ready. Heat oven to 150C/130C fan/gas 2.

Scoop the cake mix into 12 deep muffin cases (an ice-cream scoop works well), then level tops with a spoon dipped in hot water. Bake for 35-45 mins until golden and just firm to touch. A skewer inserted should come out clean. Cool on a wire rack.

Unravel the marzipan onto a work surface lightly dusted with icing sugar. Stamp out 12 rounds, 6cm across. Brush the cake tops with apricot jam, top with a marzipan round and press down lightly.Make up the fondant icing to a spreading consistency, then swirl on top of each cupcake. Decorate with sugared almonds and snowflakes, then leave to set. Will keep in a tin for 3 weeks.

Fruity ice-lolly pens

Prep:10 mins Cook:15 mins - 20 mins Easy Makes 6

Ingredients

50ml sugar-free blackcurrant cordial

50ml sugar-free orange cordial

5 tsp each red and orange natural food colouring, plus extra for painting

50g blueberry

50g strawberry, chopped

a few red grapes, halved

Directions:

Pour each cordial into a separate jug, and add the corresponding food colouring. Stir in 100ml water.

Put the blueberries, strawberries and grapes into the ice-lolly moulds and pour the blackcurrant mixture up to the brim of 3 moulds.

Pour the orange cordial into the remaining 3 moulds. Freeze for 4 hrs. 2Remove the lollies from the moulds and dot extra food colouring onto a dish.

Dip the lollies into the colouring and use to draw on clean paper– while enjoying the lolly at the same time.

Chocolate & raspberry pots

Prep:15 mins Cook:10 mins Serves 6

Ingredients

200g plain chocolate (not too bitter, 50% or less)

100g frozen raspberry, defrosted or fresh raspberries
500g Greek yogurt

3 tbsp honey

chocolate curls or sprinkles, for serving

Directions:

Break the chocolate into small pieces and place in a heatproof bowl. Bring a little water to the boil in a small saucepan, then place the bowl of chocolate on top, making sure the bottom of the bowl does not touch the water. Leave the chocolate to melt slowly over a low heat.

Remove the chocolate from the heat and leave to cool for 10 mins. Meanwhile, divide the raspberries between 6 small ramekins or glasses.

When the chocolate has cooled slightly, quickly mix in the yogurt and honey. Spoon the chocolate mixture over the raspberries. Place in the fridge to cool, then finish the pots with a few chocolate shavings before serving.

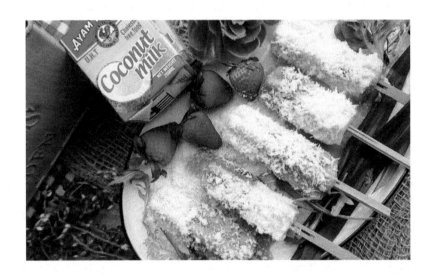

Lightning Source UK Ltd.
Milton Keynes UK
UKHW021403070521
383306UK00005B/128